Aquarius

Also by Sally Kirkman

SALLY KIRKMAN

Aquarius

The Art of Living Well and Finding
Happiness According to Your Star Sign

HODDER

First published in Great Britain in 2018 by Hodder & Stoughton
An Hachette UK company

1

A CIP catalogue record for this title is available from the British Library

Hardback ISBN 978 1 473 67663 3

Typeset in Celeste 11.5/17 pt by Palimpsest Book Production Limited,
Falkirk, Stirlingshire

Printed in the United States of America by LSC Communications

Hodder & Stoughton policy is to use papers that are natural,
renewable and recyclable products and made from wood grown in
sustainable forests. The logging and manufacturing processes are expected
to conform to the environmental regulations of the country of origin.

Hodder & Stoughton Ltd
Carmelite House
50 Victoria Embankment
London EC4Y 0DZ

www.hodder.co.uk

Contents

• • • • •

Introduction

•••••

Before computers, books or a shared language, people were fascinated by the movement of the stars and planets. They created stories and myths around them. We know that the Babylonians were one of the first people to record the zodiac, a few hundred years BC.

In ancient times, people experienced a close connection to the earth and the celestial realm. The adage 'As above, so below', that the movement of the planets and stars mirrored life on earth and human affairs, made perfect sense. Essentially, we were all one, and ancient people sought symbolic meaning in everything around them.

We are living in a very different world now, in

which scientific truth is paramount; yet many people are still seeking meaning. In a world where you have an abundance of choice, dominated by the social media culture that allows complete visibility into other people's lives, it can be hard to feel you belong or find purpose or think that the choices you are making are the right ones.

It's this calling for something more, the sense that there's a more profound truth beyond the objective and scientific, that leads people to astrology and similar disciplines that embrace a universal truth, an intuitive knowingness. Today astrology has a lot in common with spirituality, meditation, the Law of Attraction, a desire to know the cosmic order of things.

Astrology means 'language of the stars' and people today are rediscovering the usefulness of ancient wisdom. The universe is always talking to you; there are signs if you listen and the more you tune in, the more you feel guided by life. This is one of astrology's significant benefits, helping you to make sense of an increasingly unpredictable world.

Used well, astrology can guide you in making the best possible decisions in your life. It's an essential skill in your personal toolbox that enables you to navigate the ups and downs of life consciously and efficiently.

About this book

Astrology is an ancient art that helps you find meaning in the world. The majority of people to this day know their star sign, and horoscopes are growing increasingly popular in the media and online.

The modern reader understands that star signs are a helpful reference point in life. They not only offer valuable self-insight and guidance, but are indispensable when it comes to understanding other people, and living and working together in harmony.

This new and innovative pocket guide updates the ancient tradition of astrology to make it relevant and topical for today. It distils the wisdom of the star signs into an up-to-date format that's easy to read and digest, and fun and informative too. Covering a broad range of topics, it offers you insight and understanding into many different areas of your life. There are some unique sections you won't find anywhere else.

The style of the guide is geared towards you being able to maximise your strengths, so you can live well and use your knowledge of your star sign to your advantage. The more in tune you are with your zodiac sign, the higher your potential to lead a happy and fulfilled life.

The guide starts with a quick introduction to your star sign, in bullet point format. This not only reveals your star sign's ancient ruling principles, but brings astrology up-to-date, with your star sign mission, an appropriate quote for your sign and how best to describe your star sign in a tweet.

The first chapter is called 'Be True To Your Sign' and is one of the most important sections in the guide. It's a comprehensive look at all aspects of your star sign, helping define what makes you special, and explaining how the rich symbolism of your zodiac sign can reveal more about your character. For example, being born at a specific time of year and in a particular season is significant in itself.

This chapter focuses in depth on the individual attributes of your star sign in a way that's positive and uplifting. It offers a holistic view of your sign and is meant to inspire you. Within this section, you find out the reasons why your star sign traits and characteristics are unique to you.

There's a separate chapter towards the end of the guide that takes this star sign information to a new level. It's called 'Your Cosmic Gifts and Talents' and tells you what's individual about you from your star sign perspective. Most importantly, it highlights your skills and strengths, offering you clear examples of how to make the most of your natural birthright.

The guide touches on another important aspect of your star sign, in the chapters entitled 'Your Shadow Side' and 'Your Star Sign Secrets'. This reveals the potential weaknesses inherent within your star sign, and the tricks and habits you can fall into if you're not aware of them. The star sign secrets might surprise you.

There's guidance here about what you can focus on to minimise the shadow side of your star sign, and this is linked in particular to your opposite sign of the zodiac. You learn how opposing forces complement each other when you hold both ends of the spectrum, enabling them to work together.

Essentially, the art of astrology is about how to find balance in your life, to gain a sense of universal or cosmic order, so you feel in flow rather than pulled in different directions.

Other chapters in the guide provide revealing information about your love life and sex life. There are cosmic tips on how to work to your star sign strengths so you can attract and keep a fulfilling relationship, and lead a joyful sex life. There's also a guide to your love compatibility with all twelve star signs.

Career, money and prosperity is another essential section in the guide. These chapters offer you vital information on your purpose in life, and how to make the most of your potential out in the world. Your star sign skills and strengths are revealed, including what sort of job or profession suits you.

There are also helpful suggestions about what to avoid and what's not a good choice for you. There's a list of traditional careers associated with your star sign, to give you ideas about where you can excel in life if you require guidance on your future direction.

Also, there are chapters in the book on practical matters, like your health and well-being, your food and diet. These recommend the right kind of exercise for you, and how you can increase your vitality and nurture your mind, body and soul, depending on your star sign. There are individual yoga poses and tarot cards that have been carefully selected for you.

Further chapters reveal unique star sign information about your image and style. This includes whether there's a particular fashion that suits you, and how you can accentuate your look and make the most of your body.

There are even chapters that can help you decide where to go on holiday and who with, and how to decorate your home. There are some fun sections, including ideal gifts for your star sign, and ideas for films, books and music specific to your star sign.

Also, the guide has a comprehensive birthday section so you can find out which famous people share your birthday. You can discover who else is born under your star sign, people who may be your role models and whose careers or gifts you can aspire to. There are celebrity examples throughout the guide too, revealing more about the unique characteristics of your star sign.

At the end of the guide, there's a Question and Answer section, which explains the astrological terms used in the guide. It also offers answers to some general questions that often arise around astrology.

This theme is continued in a useful section entitled Additional Information. This describes the symmetry of astrology and shows you how different patterns connect the twelve star signs. If you're a beginner to astrology, this is your next stage, learning about the elements, the modes and the houses.

View this book as your blueprint, your guide to you and your future destiny. Enjoy discovering astrological revelations about you, and use this pocket guide to learn how to live well and find happiness according to your star sign.

A QUICK GUIDE TO AQUARIUS

• • • • •

Aquarius Birthdays: 21 January to 18 February

Zodiac Symbol: The Water-bearer

Ruling Planet: Saturn – traditional; Uranus – modern

Mode/Element: Fixed Air

Colour: Electric blue, neon colours

Part of the Body: Shins, ankles and circulation

Day of the Week: Saturday

Top Traits: Forward-thinking, Unique, Socially Responsible

Your Star Sign Mission: to join with

like-minded people to further goals that benefit society; to rattle the status quo

Best At: thinking outside the box, genius ideas, being a maverick, finding your tribe, backing a good cause, taking a stand, knowing your own mind, advancing the realms of knowledge

Weaknesses: easily distracted, emotionally detached, space cadet, stubborn, dogmatic, perverse

Key Phrase: I evaluate

Aquarius Quote: 'Be yourself. Embrace your quirks. Being weird is a wonderful thing.' Ed Sheeran

How to describe Aquarius in a Tweet: Hippy boho type, into new age & latest gadgets. Loves community living & social equality. Can be Spock-like, favours mental intelligence

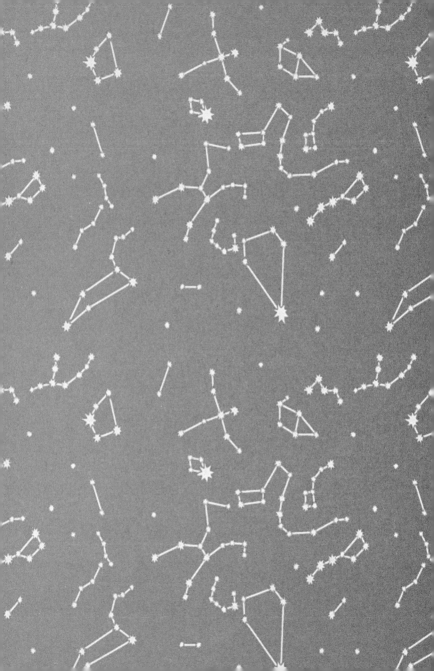

Be True To Your Sign

• • • • •

You are both a realist and an idealist, and your sign of Aquarius is an organisational genius. You straddle the old and the new with ease, reinventing structure and tradition in modern and up-to-date ways. A progressive thinker, you excel in life when you allow your innovative and original ideas free rein.

Aquarius season kicks in early every year when winter is digging in its heels in the northern hemisphere, and those New Year resolutions have either been forgotten or become a habit.

The weather is often bleak at this time, but there's nothing grey about the Aquarius character. It might still be the depths of winter, but various celebrations take place now, fittingly for a sociable Aquarius. Burns Night takes place on 25 January, Chinese New Year falls on the new moon in Aquarius season, Carnival often takes place now, depending on the dates of Easter, and Valentine's Day highlights romance on 14 February. The weather might be grim, but there are plenty of opportunities to get together with friends and be convivial and social, your birthday included.

This is in keeping with your status as one of the air signs, which are linked to networking, social get-togethers, communication and the transfer of information. Without other people in your life, you wouldn't be nearly as lively and excited about the world. You need people in your life to bounce ideas off, and to team up with to pursue joyful and rewarding mutual goals. Being on your own would be boring for the socially oriented Aquarius.

You process everything through your mind in a logical and reasoned manner. 'What do you think?'

is a better question to ask the typical Aquarius than 'How do you feel?' It's the mental and intellectual realm where you are most comfortable. You love to be informed, to impart your knowledge to others, to discuss and debate, to philosophise and learn.

Your zodiac symbol is the Water-bearer, but you're not a water sign. This wouldn't fit the Aquarius archetype because water rules the emotions, and Aquarius' response to life is first and foremost via thinking. You tend to be calm under pressure and capable of detaching yourself from your feelings when you suspect this might be more helpful or reasonable for a particular situation.

You are the Water-bearer of the zodiac because of your ability to transmit information, to pass on what you know, to filter the flow of life, to discard what's needed and preserve what's useful. You're interested in sharing ideas, finding things out, spreading knowledge and wisdom for the good of all.

Also, the sign of Aquarius rules circulation in the body, including the flow of oxygen to the lungs and bloodstream. The brain too is a busy circuit, with synapses and neutrons firing off information in intricate connections. You are the modem of the zodiac, the channel through which information flows.

Similarly, you're often at one with the modern world where the airwaves rule the skies, and global technology enables you to find things out at the click of a button and to be in touch with someone on the other side of the world instantaneously.

The typical Aquarius is progressive, modern-thinking and, very often, way ahead of their time. These themes resonate with the fact that Aquarius' modern planetary ruler is Uranus, which was discovered in 1781. The events and significant developments at the time a planet was discovered can reveal a lot about that planet's symbolism.

Uranus' discovery coincided with the French Revolution and the American War of Independence, not to mention the beginning of the Industrial Revolution. Uranus' core principles, therefore, include rebellion, individuality, freedom and liberty, new and unconventional ideas and social and technological advancement. These concepts are key themes in the Aquarius psyche.

Uranus is one of the two planets linked to Aquarius. Traditionally, your planet is Saturn, representing stability, boundaries, moderation and responsibility. Therefore, you have one foot firmly placed in tradition and the old ways, and the other foot ready to stride out into the future. You are always pushing back the boundaries of life to see how far you can go.

The role of the archetypal Aquarius is to shake things up, to be the agent of change, to be innovative and original, to champion progress and the modern way of thinking. However, you rarely break things down entirely or use violence to bring about change. Instead, you prefer to create something new from what's already established, and you choose to do so through the world of ideas and communication.

You tend to have firm principles. You're one of the fixed signs, able to hold firm for what you believe in and, when pushed to the limit, you can become dogmatic and stubborn. You don't give up easily when you believe you're on the right track.

Like all of the air signs, you are keen to play an active role in the society you live in. This is especially true for you because the sign of Aquarius rules the eleventh house in astrology, which highlights friends, groups, the collective, social organisations and political alliances. This is Aquarius' playground.

If you're a typical Aquarius, you care about world events and want to play an active role in society. Your idealistic nature means that you naturally take on a position of social responsibility, and you are often drawn towards humanitarian and environmental issues.

Wherever you want to see progress made, you will be keen not only to communicate your own thoughts and ideas but to inspire other people to get involved too.

The global village is Aquarius' stamping ground, and you see yourself as part of a wider world community. At your best, you hold true to the idea that everyone is born equal, and you will often pursue what's fair and just for the whole.

The irony of your sign is that even though you are so tightly interconnected with other people through your friendships, your community and your social and political connections, you see yourself as an outsider.

Your individual nature defines you not only in your being unique and different but also in your feeling that you don't fit in. It can take you a while to find your tribe, and even when you do so, you still prioritise your freedom, so you can walk your own path rather than follow the herd. The archetypal Aquarius is an unconventional free spirit who favours the original and eccentric.

Your Shadow Side

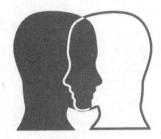

You might already have some idea about your shadow side if you are aware of or have ever been called some of the nicknames Aquarians often attract. The two most common are 'space cadet' and 'airhead', with 'weird freak' coming in a close third.

'Airhead' refers to the fact that because you get so caught up in your thoughts, and respond to everything with logic and reason, it's easy for you to disconnect. Other people see you as aloof and emotionally cool. Sometimes you disappear so far inside your own head that you haven't got a clue what's going on around you. This can be exceptionally frustrating for the people closest to you.

Modern technology hasn't helped either because it's so easy to lose yourself and lose time through the interface of a computer, phone or tablet. If you dive too deep into the virtual world, it can be hard to pull yourself back out and notice what's going on in the real world.

Worst-case scenario is that you end up with a functioning virtual life but very few friends or outside interests beyond the blur of a computer screen. This rarely makes for a fulfilled Aquarius.

Your modern ruler, Uranus, represents all things technological and contemporary and psychologically it's associated with dissociation. Therefore, inherent within every Aquarius is the ability to 'split off', to detach, to unplug.

In particular, you tend to disconnect from difficult or painful emotions, as you prefer to try to understand and rationalise them. You might be the type of Aquarius who compartmentalises emotions in their separate boxes. Sometimes you dive in to one of these boxes head first, whereas at other times you lock them tightly shut.

There are links here to the Aquarius theme of feeling like an outsider, believing that in some way you're different from other people and 'cut off' from others. It can take you a fair amount of your lifetime to recognise that being an Aquarius means you're extraordinary rather than ordinary, and that this is something to treasure rather than reject.

At its most extreme, your shadow side turns you into a robotic android, the 'Spock' of the zodiac. Then it's particularly important that you find a way to come back to yourself, to your heart, to your emotions. This is where you can learn from your opposite sign of Leo – opposite signs complement each other and have much to offer and teach each other.

The Sun mostly wants to be seen and to shine bright, and it can do so in Leo, the sign of the ego. The Sun isn't as comfortable in your sign of Aquarius as here personal ego is diminished.

When you're not in love with yourself or are disconnected from your self, you can come across as cold and heartless. Leo rules the heart, and it represents passion. When you feel alive and enthusiastic, and every synapse in your brain is switched on, then you can radiate joy back out into the world and connect on a real level.

Your Star Sign Secrets

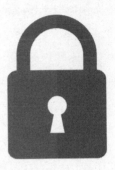

Shhh, don't tell anyone but your greatest fear is that other people are more interesting than you. You pride yourself on acquiring knowledge and being well informed. You often have a great story or anecdote to relate, you have a zany sense of humour and you like to think that you always have something to add to any conversation. You have a wealth of fascinating facts at your finger-tips and an opinion about everything. Therefore, you hate it if someone thinks you're boring or,

God forbid, you bore yourself. This is Aquarius' star sign secret.

You have another secret too, which is that you have a huge heart and an immense capacity for caring. The only problem is this doesn't always come across because you feel vulnerable wearing your heart on your sleeve and you get hurt easily. This is why you sometimes think it's safer to pretend you don't care and hide your feelings.

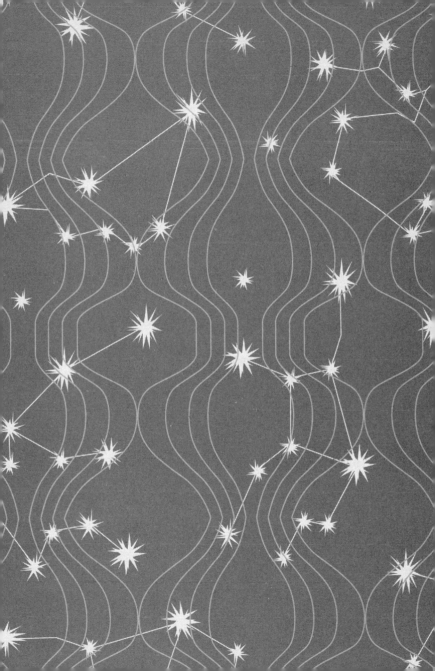

Your Love Life

Knowing about your star sign is an absolute essential when it comes to love and relationships. Once you understand what drives you, nurtures you and keeps you happy in love, then you can be true to who you are rather than try to be someone you're not.

Plus, once you recognise your weak points when it comes to relationships (and everyone has them), you can learn to moderate them and focus instead on boosting your strengths to find happiness in love.

> **KEY CONCEPTS:** dating mix-ups, love and friendship, an open relationship, love across any divide, keep the spark of love alive

Cosmic Tip: Your partner must be your best friend and your lover; only a meeting of minds will create a lasting relationship

Meeting new people is rarely a challenge for a typical Aquarius, as you are friendly and popular. You often have a varied social life and a wide circle of friends, which makes it easy for you to hook up with new people. Plus, you can be a great flirt as you take an interest in others.

Moving a compatible friendship on to a love relationship, however, isn't always that straight-forward. For starters, you are not a natural when it comes to the subtle signals of dating, and you don't always pick up on the fact that someone's attracted to you.

You too can give mixed messages, even if this isn't intentional. You blow hot and cold without realising it. For example, at a party you can talk to someone for hours late into the night, but not necessarily because you're interested in them romantically.

Similarly, you are easily distracted, and if you don't return someone's calls or you miss a date, it doesn't automatically mean that you don't want to see them again. It might just be that your attention has been diverted and, when you're not 100% plugged in, you can be forgetful.

When it comes to forming relationships too, you aren't always straight with the other person. This is because you'd rather avoid a difficult or painful conversation if you don't want to take a relationship further. Instead you cut off contact, when perhaps it would be kinder to be direct and honest.

Knowing what you want can also be a conundrum for the typical Aquarius, as you are often a mix of contradictions. Take your two ruling planets, Saturn and Uranus. Saturn requires stability and commitment, while Uranus demands freedom and variety. Put the two together, and it can mean that you want different things at different times in your life. This adds an extra challenge to finding a lasting relationship that works for you.

When it comes to finding the right person, you often start with a clean slate, and you rarely allow race, culture, religion, age or even gender to limit your love possibilities. You, more than any other star sign, can find love across any divide.

What is important to you, however, is that any potential partner fascinate you. Being with someone staid, boring or predictable is a complete no-no to the Aquarius individual.

Friendship and compatibility are absolute essentials if you want a fulfilling and long-lasting love life. If your other half isn't also your best friend, you will quickly grow bored. You need a partner who not only finds you exciting but vice versa; they must be someone who entertains and interests you.

Other factors play a significant role in Aquarius' love compatibility. One element is principles. Being with a partner who has contrasting political views to yourself, for example, will challenge your relationship. Also, you would find it hard to be with someone who exhibits racist or sexist tendencies as your natural tendency is to be fair and open-minded. An ideal partner must have a good heart and caring nature.

A definite no-no when it comes to a relationship is a partner who regularly indulges in amateur dramatics or weeping and wailing. You can entertain this kind of behaviour for a while because you do love to try to solve other people's problems. Over time, however, this would wear you down. Ideally, you want to be in a relationship that's calm the majority of the time, with a partner who's fair-minded.

Adaptability is also a fundamental concept for you when it comes to finding happiness in love. You are a freedom-lover, and even in a committed relationship, you won't take kindly to being tied down, held back or being told what to do. You are one of the signs of the zodiac who can tolerate and potentially enjoy an open relationship. Anything goes in Aquarius' world so, if it works for you, experiment with all options.

When you do find love, you always bring something different and unique to a relationship, and you want your life together to be fun and exciting. You like to keep active and be on the move and to share different interests and groups of friends with your other half.

If love is to last, treat your partner as special and make time to work at it. If you're up all night participating in online chat rooms, or you spend more time on your phone than connecting with your partner on a date or being intimate, your other half has every right to feel aggrieved.

Similarly, you'll get fed up if your partner puts their feet up in front of the TV every night. You hate to get stuck in a rut, and your ideal relationship is one in which there's equality but also an extra spark of added excitement. You want and need a partner to bring something extra to your life. In return, they will receive a witty, educated and provocative life partner, even if sometimes you leave most of the relationship decisions up to them.

Connect with your heart too, because love is dull without a heart connection. As an Aquarius, break-ups often affect you badly, and you're likely to batten down the hatches around your heart so as not to be hurt again. Without the willingness to be vulnerable, however, a relationship can't deepen, and love won't flourish. Self-protection is a sensible approach, but don't let the enjoyment of love pass you by.

Your Love Matches

Some star signs are a better love match for you than others. The classic combinations are the other two star signs from the same element as your sign, air; in Aquarius' case, Gemini and Libra.

The only danger with the air signs is that you end up becoming best mates, but you lose the spark and excitement of an intimate love relationship. It can become too cerebral, and you can forget the physical. You need a partner who reminds you of the importance of a deep connection when it comes to love.

It's also important to recognise that any star sign match can be a good match if you're willing to learn from each other and use astrological insight to understand more about what makes the other person tick. Here's a quick guide to your love matches with all twelve star signs:

Aquarius–Aries: Sexy Sextiles

You two are the white knights of the zodiac, and a mutual love of social, environmental or humanitarian concerns draws you close. You share a passion for the new, but if your relationship is to survive into the future, you need to reinvent and renew your love always.

Aquarius–Taurus: Squaring Up To Each Other

If you're more like your traditional ruler Saturn, you are the archetypal business owner who will cater for this sign's creature comforts. More like modern ruler Uranus, and you are a breath of fresh air to the routine-loving Taurus. It's through your differences that you learn to appreciate and understand each other better.

Aquarius–Gemini: In Your Element

You two have a lot in common, but it's going to take something special to move your friendship on to being a loving relationship. An open relationship is a strong possibility, and a wide circle of friends is a given. If you do go your separate ways, your friendship will last the test of time.

Aquarius–Cancer: Soulmates

You are logical, and Cancer is emotional which may seem like an odd match, but this pairing can work. You love to solve problems, while Cancer worries for England, the perfect match. If you both want the relationship to work, there's plenty to keep the two of you interested.

Aquarius–Leo: Opposites Attract

Aquarius is cerebral, more introvert than Leo and interested in the group and social dynamic, but with a wacky side. Leo is a natural extrovert who loves to perform and adores a life filled with play and a chance to be self-expressive. Two unique individuals who can be best friends.

Aquarius–Virgo: Soulmates

Your sign meets Virgo on an intellectual plane. As two of the most intelligent and studious signs of the zodiac, you can be best friends as well as lovers. That you share an interest in social and environmental concerns helps keep the spark of love alive.

Aquarius–Libra: In Your Element

This combination pits the individual (Aquarius) with the romantic (Libra). That's not to say that you don't love being in a relationship but you need your freedom. You keep the connection alive when you deepen your love within the realm of the weird or unconventional.

Aquarius–Scorpio: Squaring Up To Each Other

The two of you together can go on a magical mystery tour and discover places that other people don't even know. At its best, you and the Scorpio in this relationship connect at a deep level, as you are both interested in pushing back the boundaries of knowledge and experience.

Aquarius–Sagittarius: Sexy Sextiles

You are the freedom lovers of the zodiac and want to roam far and wide and live life to the full. Commitment is the C-word that neither sign is comfortable with, so there needs to be a broader purpose or reason to stay together for ever. An open relationship suits this combination best.

Aquarius–Capricorn: Next-Door Neighbours

Your sign and Capricorn are both Saturn-ruled, and you are at your best out in the world. You hoard friends like Capricorn hoards trophies, and Capricorn can be too stuffy for your non-conformist ways. The stereotypical 'odd' match that proves that, in love, anything goes.

Aquarius–Aquarius: Two Peas In A Pod

This is a meeting of minds and a genuinely original combination. Unconventional and eccentric, you both love to shock, and you need a partner who's not afraid to be a rebel. Whether you're into alternative health or social concerns, you thrive when pursuing shared beliefs.

Aquarius–Pisces: Next-Door Neighbours

Aquarius and Pisces are both hippies at heart, and an unconventional love affair appeals to you both. You can be too emotionally detached for sensitive Pisces, who weeps at the drop of a hat. If you learn to love each other's differences, you can go the full distance in love.

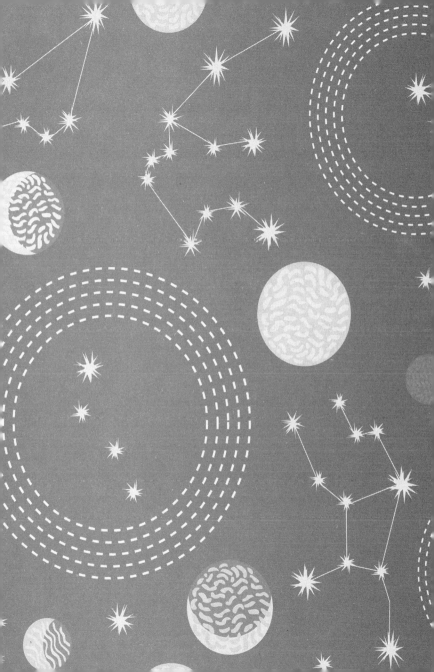

Your Sex Life

• • • • •

There is a side to the Aquarius character that's akin to the hippy culture of the 60s. This is especially true if you lean more towards the unique and outrageous character of your modern ruler Uranus.

Sexual liberation and free love are fundamental to the 60s vibe, and you too might go through a phase in life where you're happy to experiment sexually, defying convention. In fact, some Aquarian lovers spend their whole existence freewheeling their way through life and love.

There are a few reasons why this approach to sex works for your sign. First, you like to be an expert at whatever you turn your hand to and second, when it comes to sexual relationships, you're keen to master any technique going.

You want not only to read up on all possible sexual positions but to be able to put them into practice. Find the right sexual partner/s, and you can be quite happy exploring and learning along the way.

Also, there is a side to your Aquarius nature that wants and needs freedom in your life. Therefore, until you're ready to settle down, you might prefer to keep sex and love separate. This is rarely difficult for you, because of your ability to detach from your emotions when necessary.

In fact, you are one of the signs of the zodiac who could easily have more than one lover on the go and, if no commitment has been agreed, find the arrangement agreeable.

For you, sex is an area of life where you believe that people should be free to make up their own minds about what they want and need, and what gives them pleasure, yourself included. It's your right to choose whether you want lots of sex or no sex at all that's imperative for the classic Aquarius. In this respect, you're sex-positive.

Feminism is attributed to your ruling planet Uranus too, because it's about the equality of the sexes. A typical Aquarius will be of the opinion that there doesn't need to be a defining role for men or women when it comes to sex, which can open up all kinds of possibilities.

You do have something of a reputation for being one of the kinkiest players of the zodiac because you're often willing to try anything that's new and exciting. Usually, you love games in the bedroom, and you'll encourage your partner to act out sexual fantasies that thrill you both.

Whether you're swinging from the chandelier or you're entwined with your partner in the lotus position, sex with you is rarely dull. If you've not yet joined the mile-high club, add it your list of exciting things to do.

There's even been a couple who've had sex while skydiving, which would thrill the wild, adventure-seeking side of your Aquarius nature. Add to this the fact that your ruler Uranus rules planes and was a sky god in mythology and you can see the attraction.

Webcam sex can be an exciting alternative if you and the one you want are miles apart. This is when being a technology geek comes into its own. Take your Aquarius credentials to the extreme, and you could even contemplate a hyperrealistic blow-up love doll as an experiment.

AQUARIUS ON A FIRST DATE

- you get distracted and arrive late

- you wear something that makes you feel special

- you end up eating little and talking lots

- you want to find out everything about your date

- you have to respond to a phone message, at least once

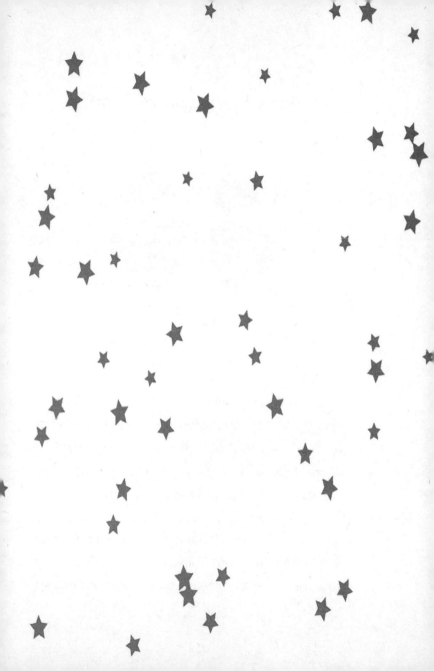

Your Friends and Family

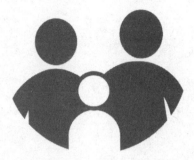

If any of the star signs of the zodiac is to have a wide and varied social life, it's Aquarius. In fact, your friendships and close connections are your lifeblood. You feed off other people, and you will always choose a night out with some of your favourite friends over being home alone.

Fun is one reason why you want to meet up with people you like and make new friends. As an Aquarius, you often have a crazy sense of humour that's madcap and original and, if you're a typical Aquarius, you see the funny side of life.

You are also a night owl, and you can happily stay up all night at a party talking to friends or take a phone call at midnight, chat for hours and still go to work looking fresh as a daisy. Socialising is one of your favourite things to do, and you will often change your plans at the drop of a hat if you receive a last-minute invitation to a fun get-together.

You also need people in your life for discussion and debate, and you're rarely interested in people who are superficial or prioritise looks over person-ality. It's a person's mind that grabs your attention, and you're drawn towards people who add some-thing special to your life.

If your friends are slightly wacky, so much the better. You'd rather hang out with people who are original and authentic than anyone who believes they have to change their personality to fit in.

When it comes to talking, there's no subject under the sun that you don't have an opinion about and which you're happy to engage in. Whatever the topic, you'll be keen to pitch in. What delights you most in life is to give other people information, sometimes whether they want to hear it or not!

If you're a typical Aquarius, you'll be interested in all things weird and wonderful, whether your particular gig is quantum science, aliens and UFOs or new age talks and workshops. Find your tribe in life, and you will have like-minded friends who get who you are and with whom you can enjoy your specialist or unique interests.

There is something of a conundrum about your sign of Aquarius and your two co-rulers; they turn you into a shy extrovert. You like people, but it can take you a while to learn how to open up and connect on a deeper level.

Friends are great, however, for teaching you about intimacy and affection. If you're a typical Aquarius, you can be the most awkward hugger at first, with both sexes, until you get used to physical contact.

You like to ask friends' advice too but, as a fixed sign, you tend to have very set opinions, and you know what you believe is right and wrong. Whatever other people say, you'll still make up your own mind and not be easily swayed by their opinions.

This is where your stubborn side kicks in, and you can dig in your heels around friendship issues. If someone wrongs you or misbehaves in your eyes, that can be enough to end the friendship, at least until your tolerant nature wins through.

When it comes to family, you're at your best meeting up for social and fun get-togethers. However, you don't find it difficult to cut ties with your family and move on with your own life.

That's not to say you won't enjoy getting together if you feel part of the family, and the bigger the celebration or family meet-up, the better. If you view your family as part of your tribe, then you'll be more than happy to play your part in family events, although sometimes your sign takes on the archetypal 'black sheep' role.

When it comes to parenting, not every Aquarius chooses to go down the route of having children, and there are different reasons for this. Firstly, with parenting comes responsibility, and you might prefer to avoid a situation in life that stymies your freedom.

Secondly, you may have strong beliefs about population control or not want to bring a child into a world where the future is uncertain. This is where your rational mind can kick in and govern your life choices.

Thirdly, you sometimes forget to have children! Seriously, this might sound odd but it does often take intention and commitment to have a child, and you might be too busy with other life plans.

The single life and solo adventures can both appeal to you as an Aquarius. Primarily, you live to the beat of your own drum, and whatever life you choose, it has to suit who you are to a T.

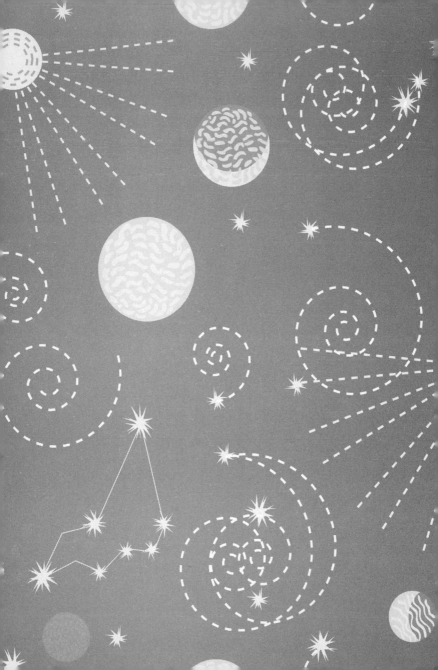

Your Health and Well-Being

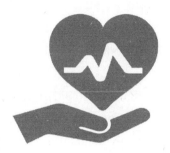

KEY CONCEPTS: exercise that's fun and social, the calming breath, medical self-diagnosis, experimental diets

Health and exercise are rarely top of Aquarius' list of priorities. Instead, you're usually more interested in cerebral activities than going to the gym. In fact, if you're a typical Aquarius, you might be of the firm belief that regular exercise is one of the most boring things you can do.

That being said, it is essential to factor some form of exercise into your routine and walking is one of the best activities for airy Aquarius. Your sign rules the ankles and walking not only strengthens them but can help improve your circulation, another area of the body ruled by Aquarius.

Get out and about in the fresh air, Aquarius' element, and breathe it in. Being one of the air signs, you can be hyper, with an overactive nervous system, so any form of meditation or mindfulness is helpful for you, to slow you down and keep you calm.

Ensure that you learn to express your feelings too and don't bottle them up. Your element of air needs to move, otherwise it becomes stagnant, and this is worth implementing on both an inner and an outer level. Allow your feelings and breath to flow and move your body.

T'ai chi is an excellent addition to the Aquarius fitness schedule. It's good for muscle strength and balance, and done on a regular basis it can have a calming effect on the body, lowering the blood pressure and keeping your heart healthy. Cycling too is another way to stay fit and do your bit to help the environment.

It is vital as an Aquarius that you look after your health. In astrology, the Sun rules vitality, but it's not as strong in your sign as it is in some other signs. Therefore, doing whatever you can to optimise your health is a sound plan and a wise investment in your future.

Join in a sports activity that is social or fun, as this will assist you in turning up week in, week out. This might include dance, especially tango, or snow sports, e.g. skiing or ice-skating. Both activities can help to strengthen your Aquarius ankles.

If you're a typical Aquarius, you actually enjoy the cold, and sometimes you prefer heading to a wintry wonderland rather than be in tropical climes. Your internal temperature gauge can veer towards cool if you experience circulation problems. You might have permanently cold feet or hands or need to wrap up more than other people.

When it comes to looking after your health, you often flip between taking conventional medical advice and experimenting with alternative treatments. Usually you like to conduct your own research, as you want to be as informed as possible about any ailments or how best to treat them. You can spend hours on the internet, finding out about new drugs and supplements until you're an expert in a particular area.

Add to this the fact that you are both rebellious and stubborn and, on some level, you're unlikely to listen to general advice and will go ahead and do your own thing anyway. This means you can end up making some unusual choices in your life when it comes to optimising your health and well-being.

The classic Aquarius has a sanguine temperament, and you often see the funny side of life. You rarely let any setbacks get you down, but instead, your comic and zany sense of humour kicks in to lift your spirits. As Lord Byron (22 January) reportedly said, 'Always laugh when you can. It is cheap medicine.'

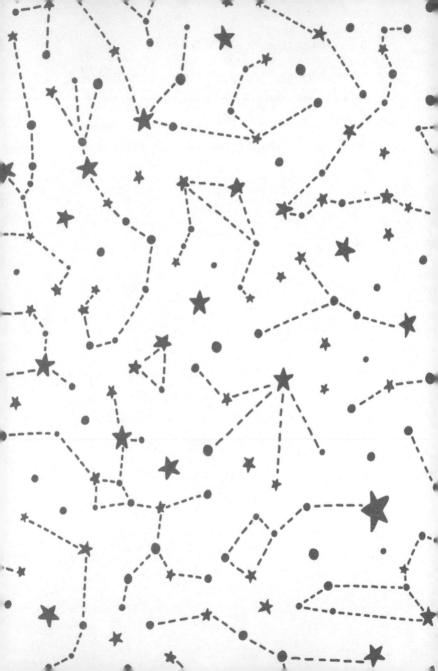

Aquarius and Food

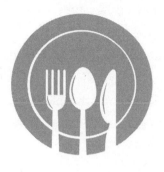

A typical Aquarius' attitude towards food and diet is often experimental, and you are open to trying anything. You like to think of yourself as a citizen of the world, and your original palate makes you the perfect candidate for sampling cuisine from as many different nations as possible.

You can swing between extremes, however, when it comes to your diet, and your unconventional approach to life extends to your eating habits as well. You can sometimes be a finicky eater and will sometimes try out weird and unusual combinations. You might experiment with a macrobiotic diet or eliminate certain foods from your cooking.

One day, you could choose to spend a fortune buying all your ingredients from an expensive health food shop, but the next day, you're back in the fast food outlets and not bothered about healthy eating at all.

You do have to watch that your extreme approach to food and diet doesn't adversely affect your system. If you start to worry too much about what you're eating, this can breed neurosis and have an adverse effect on you. Cutting back on stimulants such as caffeine can be a good idea for you, especially if you drink lots of coffee to keep you buzzing.

Light foods tend to suit you best rather than a diet that's rich or heavy; this will aid your digestion. Lots of colour and vibrancy in the look of your food stimulates your appetite, so ensure that you have plenty of fruit and salad on the table during mealtimes. The more you enjoy your diet and what you eat, the more balanced and relaxed you feel inside.

In restaurants, you favour a modern setting, especially if hi-tech gadgets are employed. Pop-up restaurants can appeal to the side of your Aquarius nature that loves immediacy and one-off experiences.

If you have strong views about animal welfare, you might choose to go vegetarian or vegan. It's not primarily about the health benefits either, but usually a matter of principle.

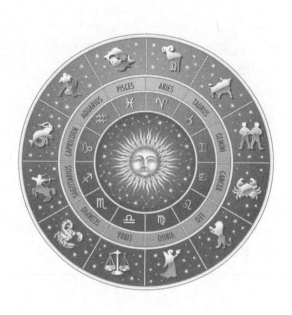

Do You Look Like An Aquarius?

People often notice you as an Aquarius because you walk either with your head in a phone or your head in the clouds. You can seem other-worldly at times and strangely disconnected from what's going on around you. That's not to say you don't come across as friendly and approachable, certainly with people you know. Some people think you're aloof, but that's more to do with your busy mind, which is always thinking.

The 'anything goes' Aquarius feature also applies to the way you look. If you lean more towards your modern ruler Uranus, you might be unusually tall or small. You also often have youthful good looks and something of the Pre-Raphaelite style about you.

The typical Aquarius complexion is pale, with a strong facial bone structure and chiselled jaw. You have distinctive eyes, dreamy and vague, and they can be a bright blue, one of Aquarius' key colours. Your hair often adds a slightly zany or bohemian element.

Your Style and Image

You are rarely interested in the latest fashions. Instead, as the holder of one of the zodiac's most unusual and eccentric signs, you dress the way you think. If you're a geek, clothes tend to be functional rather than stylish, and the classic Aquarius look is always your own. If anyone can mix and match styles and eras, it's Aquarius.

The space-age, futuristic look suits the more way-out Aquarius, but if any era is said to define you, it's the hippy days of the 60s. This was your period in fashion as you became the sign of the moment when young people everywhere were singing along to 'The Age of Aquarius' from the musical *Hair* (1967). Dubbed the American Tribal Love-Rock Musical, *Hair* was a celebration of the hippy culture and the sexual revolution of the era. The musical ended with all the cast completely naked.

Mary Quant (11 February) was *the* fashion designer of the 60s. Her style creations were the miniskirt and hot pants, and she put the fun back into fashion. The decade was a time of vivid colour, tie-dye materials, neon colours and electric blue, all critical components of Aquarius' colour palette.

There are no limits to what you can pull off in the style department; hair or clothes, accessories or make-up – so if you want to go colourful, outrageous and over the top, do it. This is one way for you to break the rules, defy convention and use your body and outfits to shock and awaken the rest of society.

The androgynous look suits you too and, like all the air signs, you can dress as boy or girl, irrespective of your sex. Your look is often gender-fluid; Aquarius women look great in men's suits with short, slicked-back hair and some Aquarius men, like Eddie Izzard (7 February), favour cross-dressing.

One of the most versatile fashion items is the legging. The revival of the legging in the modern day is credited to eccentric Aquarius costume designer Patricia Field (12 February). Field has been called 'one of fashion's greatest visionaries', fitting for the Aquarius archetype. Whatever you choose to wear, make it your own. Your Aquarius birthright is to stand out from the crowd.

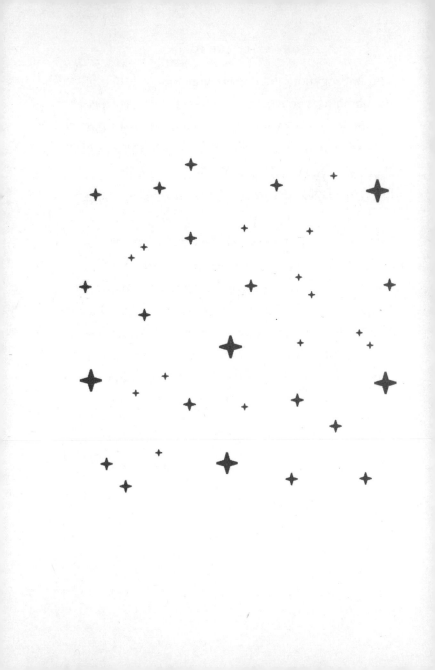

Your Home

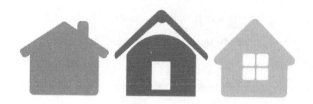

Your Ideal Aquarius Home:

An eco-friendly home, whether you go for a solar roof and produce your own energy, build your home into a hill with locally sourced materials or champion urban gardening with a roof garden or community allotment.

As an Aquarius, you need freedom and space in your life, so a home that fits these criteria is ideal for you. Somewhere spacious with low furniture and little clutter is the typical Aquarius model.

It depends too what the function of your home is; whether it's a place to rest your head, or you want a space where you can invite friends round to socialise, play games and hang out together. You are rarely materialistic, and a typical Aquarius isn't interested in designer gear or status symbols.

In fact, you are often not attached to the traditional concept of what a home means. You can happily make somewhere new your home, but you rarely invest your emotions into the place you live.

In general, new styles and trends appeal to you more than old furniture or antiques. If you're a typical Aquarius, you might prefer to invest in new technology and gadgets, rather than furnishings: state-of-the-art home automation that controls the appliances, music system, lights and heating at the touch of a button.

Your sign can take decorating to the extreme too, and it's often a case of 'anything goes'. Diagonal lines and zigzag wallpaper? Yes, of course. A chrome and glass table, a lime green sofa in a modern style, steel units in the kitchen? Why not.

Vibrant colours dictate the Aquarius palette, and you can choose from electric blue, silver, neon colours and any shade that's futuristic and modern. Add splashes of colour to a more neutral background for a distinctive look.

Contemporary materials, such as vinyl, plastic or aluminium, often appeal to your modern taste, or weird and wonderful objects and abstract art. Two Aquarius artists who give you a sense of what is an archetypal Aquarius look are Jackson Pollock (28 January) and Jeff Koons (21 January). Sometimes you enjoy art for its shock value, more so than for any soothing or appealing effects.

Retro household items that have come back into fashion also entertain your Aquarius love of quirkiness or kitsch. A lava lamp, for example – this is the sort of unusual piece that you love if you're a typically eccentric Aquarius.

If that sounds too way-out for you, then go down the IKEA route; Sweden as a country is associated with your sign. Again the focus is on modern living. IKEA's website states that one way to describe their home furnishing style is to describe nature – 'full of light and fresh air, restrained yet unpretentious.' That sounds like an ideal arrangement for an Aquarius home.

Ultimately, however, Aquarius is the sign of the individual, which means that one style of home does not suit all. You might choose community living, which suits your egalitarian nature, be entirely comfortable in a studio flat, house-sit your way around the world or bid for a pod on a space station. The ideal Aquarius home is unique to you.

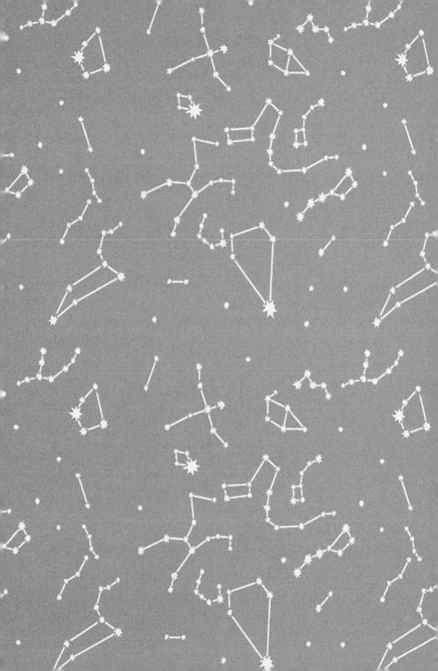

Your Star Sign Destinations

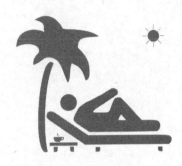

IDEAS FOR AQUARIUS:

- *visit a remote tribe*

- *take a tour of the space station at NASA*

- *attend a Pride event anywhere in the world*

Did you know that many cities and countries are ruled by a particular star sign? This is based on when a country was founded, although sometimes, depending on their history, places have more than one star sign attributed to them.

This can help you decide where to go on holiday, and it can also explain why there are certain places where you feel at home straight away.

Your individual approach to life often extends to trips away. You are rarely someone who wants to go and sit on a beach or head for the obvious holiday hotspots. Instead, a holiday suits you best when it has a purpose, e.g. a study break or a chance to learn a new skill.

Also, you like to see where life leads you and if there's a story behind a trip, this appeals to your spontaneous nature. You might meet someone on a night out, for example, who relates a weird and wonderful experience and invites you to visit them or take a trip together. If it's unrepeatable and different, it has the Aquarius signature written all over it.

81

You're also one of the star signs who can be happy travelling on your own and going solo is often your style. You might be keen to visit friends who live around the world who you've met on- or offline, so you get to experience a country or city from the perspective of a local.

If you're an Aquarius geek, you could have a specific reason to visit a country or city, whether there's a museum that you want to see or you want to further your knowledge and interests.

Charity work can be another good reason for travelling, and taps into your humanitarian side. If you have the time and money, you could be one of the first people to leap on a plane and help as an aid worker after a natural disaster.

Talking of planes, as a typical Aquarius you are usually well informed about your carbon footprint. This might lead you to spend longer in one place than a typical fortnight's holiday, or even choose to live abroad.

Mostly, the Aquarius traveller rarely wants to go where everyone else is heading, but instead prefers to line up a real adventure or immerse themself in the local culture.

Countries ruled by Aquarius include Russia, Sweden, Iran, Finland, Sri Lanka

Cities ruled by Aquarius include Brighton in the UK; Moscow and St Petersburg in Russia; Hamburg, Bremen and Ingolstadt in Germany

Your Career and Vocation

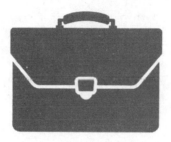

> **KEY CONCEPTS:** science buff/computer nerd, making the world a better place, freedom and flexibility, objective thinking

Any career you enter into has to stimulate your mind. You want a job or role that will challenge your thought processes, a profession into which it's worth investing your time and energy. Aquarius is fixed air, so you not only have an intelligent mind (air) but you can concentrate (fixed) too.

You look at things objectively, and a career that involves evaluation, assessment and research fits the Aquarius archetype. You like to push the boundaries of knowledge, and you're more suited to a career that's progressive, rather than anything overly traditional.

A tedious nine-to-five job won't hold your attention for long unless you can put your skills of innovation and invention to good use. The fields of science and technology are often a popular choice for the Aquarius employee.

This is where you can combine the skill sets of your co-rulers, Saturn and Uranus. Saturn lends you organisational ability, and Uranus turns your gaze towards the future. If you're a typically tech-savvy Aquarius, you could do well in the world of computers, engineering or space travel.

Going places no one has gone before and discovering new concepts and ideas, and scientific or technological breakthroughs, can be the ultimate dream for the classic Aquarius.

You're best working in a friendly and cooperative environment, and you make a favourite member of any team. You're sociable, and you can usually work out how to avoid getting wound up by the most demanding person in the office. In this situation, you do what's necessary to fit in, and you rarely rise to drama or get involved in petty office politics.

You're not primarily drawn to one-to-one type relationships within a career context. If anything, you prefer not to become too personal with colleagues or clients, although you're fundamentally friendly and fun to work with.

Authority can be a stumbling block, however, as you don't take kindly to being told what to do, which can be a challenge as an employee. You hate to be restricted and, therefore, a job that allows you freedom and flexibility is ideal for your independent Aquarius nature.

You often excel in a career that furthers society or supports a charitable cause. This can be more of a vocation for you than a career plan, and money is rarely the primary motivation for you in any profession. You would much rather be doing a job that's worthwhile and where you can make a difference than just raking in the cash.

You fit well into organisations where you can team up with other people to take on a public-spirited role. This might be within the community or society, or as part of a political, humanitarian or environmental goal.

Working alongside other people towards a better world ticks many boxes for your altruistic nature. If you're a typical Aquarius, you believe in the principles of liberty and equality, and you often choose a career where you can defend other people and champion the underdog.

You are the experimentalist of the zodiac too, so find your niche, the one thing you're good at that's new to other people, and promote the socks off it. If anyone's going to be a whizz at internet marketing, can use social media to generate interest and take a product or concept viral, it's Aquarius #geniusidea.

Many companies and organisations are looking for people with new business strategies who have their finger on the pulse of today, so keep up to date with what's happening in the world of work. You have a natural ability to sniff out new trends, even in an established business.

You often love the crazy, the wacky, the weird and new age thinking, and the self-help industry calls strongly to your inner hippy. Whether you're keen to promote community living, eco-homes, vegan food or clothing, or you want to save the whale, save trees or save the world; there's a cause with your name written on it.

It might not propel you up the career ladder, but you'll have a blast defending your principles and playing your part in something you believe in.

Solo missions appeal to your Aquarius nature, and you don't have to team up with other people to gain fulfilment in life. Take Charles Lindbergh (4 February), who was the first person to fly solo across the Atlantic.

If your free-spirited nature wants to roam, choose your dream goal and work towards it. Sometimes in a corporate or traditional work environment, you feel hemmed in and begin to develop conformist and herd-like tendencies.

This is often the time to activate your inner rebel, so you can break out and unleash your Aquarius genius. You have top star sign credentials to create something in your life that you're remembered for.

If you're seeking inspiration for a new job, take a look at the list below, which reveals the careers that traditionally come under the Aquarius archetype:

TRADITIONAL AQUARIUS CAREERS

IT specialist

scientist

engineer

games inventor

astronaut

airline pilot

astrologer

meteorologist

sociologist

social worker

charity fundraiser

website designer

brand ambassador

social media expert

marketing strategist

online business owner

vlogger

conceptual artist
science fiction writer
political activist

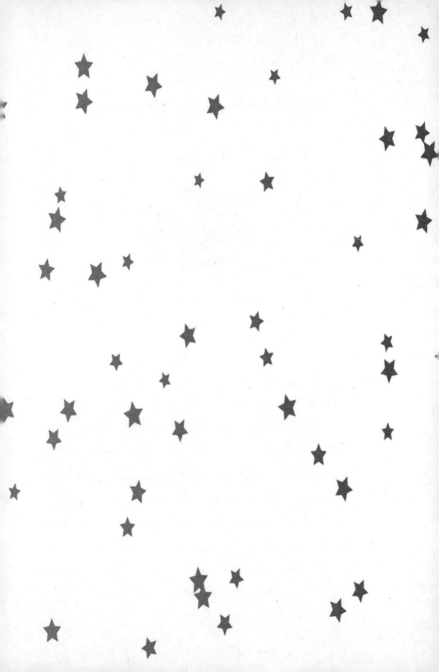

Your Money and Prosperity

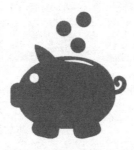

It's rare to find an Aquarius whose primary goal in life is to create wealth. In fact, you are usually someone who considers the trappings of big money sordid or at least not significant. You scarcely ever meet a flashy Aquarius, dripping in bling and with status symbols to match.

Also, money is often a dirty word to you if you associate money with greed, big business and corporate multinationals. You're a principled character, and you're more likely to believe in the fair distribution of wealth than in making the rich richer and the poor poorer.

Even if you become hugely successful in life and wealth is a by-product of your triumph, you're unlikely to flaunt your riches. Instead, you often prefer to share your good fortune. You might choose to plough your money back into society or pledge a percentage of your wealth to philanthropic causes.

The typical Aquarius is savvy when it comes to money and investing. This is where your cool and calm demeanour and your objective, reasoning faculties come into their own. There's rarely an emotional connection for you concerning money, which means you can make rational and smart decisions.

Also, one of your skills is spotting new trends, and in this respect you're the zodiac's fortune teller. Your talent at research combined with your futuristic gaze means you have an excellent ability to play the stock market and invest wisely.

What you're not so brilliant at is paying close attention to facts and figures. You often have great ideas and enthusiasm, but you're not always 100% reliable. Also, you can go off on a tangent and forget, for example, to check when an interest rate is coming to an end.

If this rings a bell and you know you have a forgetful or scatty side to your nature, team up with someone who has complementary skills to your own. The earth signs, Taurus, Virgo and Capricorn, are extremely thorough at the nuts-and-bolts end of money management.

Getting yourself a good accountant or financial adviser can also be a helpful move, especially if you are the type of Aquarius who isn't that bothered about money and wealth.

Security does matter to you, however, more than other people think. You like to have something tangible for your efforts, whether you buy a home and rent it out while you're travelling, or look at other ways to use property as a means to pursue personal gain.

Having a solid backup in your life that you can rely on minimises sleepless nights worrying about money. You are usually uncomfortable borrowing money too, and would rather be financially self-sufficient. As long as you have enough to get by and you don't run up massive debts, that can feel like plenty for the classic Aquarius.

You're not going to be impressed by a big bank account, but you are influenced by how other people use their money, whether they make smart investments or contribute to charity. If you can use money to make money and subsequently make a difference in the world, that's the Aquarius money dream.

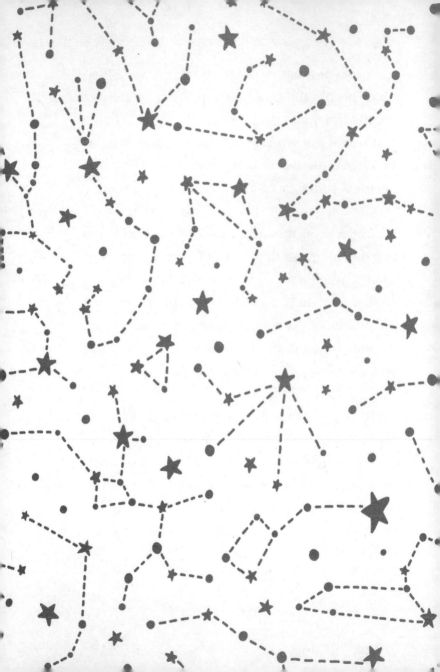

Your Cosmic Gifts and Talents

Famous Quirks

As an Aquarius, you rarely seek out fame; instead, fame finds you. Ed Sheeran (17 February) describes himself as 'a really geeky ginger kid with spectacles and a massive guitar', and he's become one of the biggest stars around. You attract fame your way, and you don't have to take a conventional route to stardom. You can take on unique roles in life and win.

Think of the brilliant actor John Hurt (22 January), known for playing iconic parts in many classic movies: among many others, the Elephant Man Joseph Merrick, Quentin Crisp in *The Naked Civil Servant* and *Alien* with its unforgettable death scene. Aquarius sports stars have their idiosyncratic talents too, which make them stand out from the crowd: there is footballer Peter Crouch (30 January) and his robot dance, and tennis player John 'You cannot be serious' McEnroe (16 February). Become famous for your quirks.

Rebel with a Cause

It was an Aquarius, James Dean (8 February), who hit cult status in the movie *Rebel Without A Cause* (1956). As an Aquarius, you are the iconoclast of the zodiac, always ready to shake things up, to question what's established and conventional, to push back the boundaries. The world needs more rebels, an appropriate role for your sign. Ideally, you will channel your rebellious instincts into a good cause rather than go off-piste without one.

Group Motivator

You're not like Leo, who is often instrumental in starting a new group or bringing people together, but what you are skilled at is taking on a significant role within a group. In fact, once you're among a group of like-minded people, you come into your own. You are fair-minded and want the best for everyone. You understand group dynamics too and know instinctively how to get everyone working together towards a common goal. Your persuasive abilities are inspiring, a fundamental characteristic of all the air signs. To 'inspire' means to breathe in, so use your breath, your voice, in a group context.

Genius Potential

To be a genius, you need to have both brilliance and dedication and thanks to your co-rulers, Saturn and Uranus, you can harness both. You're a practical (Saturn) visionary (Uranus).

A classic example is Wolfgang Amadeus Mozart (27 January), who was prodigiously talented and made music from the age of five. He died young but still managed to compose more than 600 works. If you allow yourself to dream *and* put in the work, you have a great chance to let your Aquarius genius shine through.

Social Activist

You are the right-on, politically correct member of the zodiac and you excel in life when you find your thing and stand up for what you believe in. The classic Aquarius example is one of the most influential women in the world, Oprah Winfrey (29 January), who overcame adversity in her own life to become a benefactor to millions of people. Whether you're a peace activist, a political activist, a grassroots activist or a green activist, if you believe in something strongly enough, your Aquarius credentials are designed to make it happen.

Be An Inventor

You are always one step ahead of the rest with your gaze firmly fixed on the future. The world of the new is Aquarius' territory. Thomas Edison (11 February) has been described as America's greatest inventor, most famous for inventing the light bulb. Another excellent example is naturalist Charles Darwin (12 February), who is renowned for his contribution to the science of evolution. Be an Aquarius inventor.

Embrace Your Weird

The world would be a less colourful and dull place without Aquarius to liven things up. You thrive as an individual when you realise the joy in being different and unique. As a child, this can be an onerous burden to carry, and you have to learn to build up your ego, to strengthen your inner confidence. It can be hard to be the weird one and not fit in. As an adult, you come into your own when you fully embrace your eccentricity, your originality. You enhance your life and the lives of others when you fully and completely embrace your weird. Dare to be different.

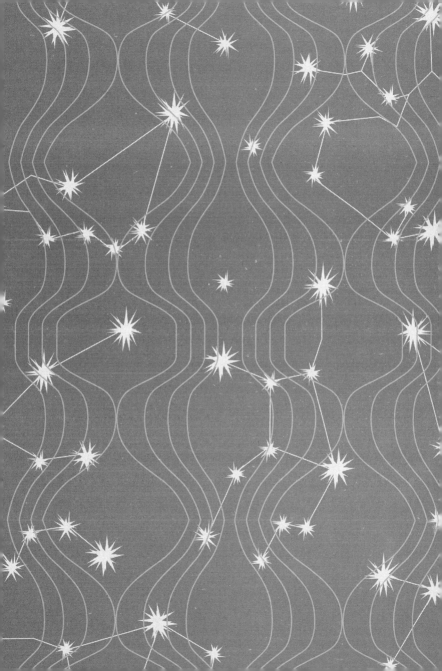

Films, Books, Music

• • • • •

Films: Science fiction and fantasy, e.g. *Avatar, Star Wars, Alien*; or *Butch Cassidy And The Sundance Kid*, starring the 'opposites attract' double act Aquarius Paul Newman (26 January) and Leo Robert Redford.

Books: *Naked Lunch* by William Burroughs (5 February), *Beloved* by Toni Morrison (18 February) or *The Color Purple* by Alice Walker (9 February).

Music: 'The Girl from Ipanema' by Stan Getz (2 February) or anti-establishment anthem 'God Save The Queen' by the Sex Pistols, fronted by John Lydon, aka Johnny Rotten (31 January).

YOGA POSE:

Chair: strengthens ankles and calves,
opens the diaphragm

TAROT CARD:

The Star

GIFTS TO BUY AN AQUARIUS:

- periodic table shower curtain
- temporary tattoos
- water jug
- wireless headphones
- astrology gift report
- Glastonbury festival ticket
- telescope
- robot butler
- electric car
- Star Gift – private jet

Aquarius Celebrities Born On Your Birthday

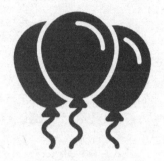

JANUARY

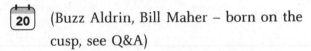

20 (Buzz Aldrin, Bill Maher – born on the cusp, see Q&A)

21 Christian Dior, Telly Savalas, Jeff Koons, Benny Hill, Placido Domingo, Martin Shaw, Geena Davis, Emma Bunton, Booboo Stewart, Sasha Pivovarova

22 Claire Rayner, Jim Jarmusch, John Hurt, Malcolm McLaren, Linda Blair, Michael Hutchence, Diane Lane, Logic

23 Django Reinhardt, Jeanne Moreau, Paula Hamilton, Tiffani Thiessen, Mistah F.A.B., Doutzen Kroes

24 Ernest Borgnine, Neil Diamond, Nastassja Kinski, John Belushi, Sharon Tate, Adrian Edmondson, Vic Reeves, Mischa Barton, Rick Salomon, Jools Holland

25 Virginia Woolf, Etta James, Alicia Keys

26 Paul Newman, Ellen DeGeneres

27 Wolfgang Amadeus Mozart, Lewis Carroll, Bridget Fonda, Rosamund Pike

28 Jackson Pollock, Alan Alda, Nicolas Sarkozy, Sarah McLachlan, Frank Skinner, Elijah Wood, J. Cole, Nick Carter, Rakim

29 Germaine Greer, Tom Selleck, Oprah Winfrey, Heather Graham, Clare Balding, Adam Lambert, Isabel Lucas

30 Franklin D. Roosevelt, Saul Alinsky, Gene Hackman, Vanessa Redgrave, Phil Collins, Christian Bale, Wilmer Valderrama, Olivia Colman, Jemima Goldsmith, Romesh Ranganathan

31 Tallulah Bankhead, Carol Channing, Norman Mailer, John Lydon, Minnie Driver, Jonathan Banks, Justin Timberlake, Portia de Rossi, Philip Glass, Kerry Washington

FEBRUARY

1 Clark Gable, Terry Jones, Princess Stephanie, Lisa Marie Presley, Brandon Lee, Harry Styles

2 Ayn Rand, James Joyce, Stan Getz, David Jason, Farrah Fawcett, Christie Brinkley, Seth Green, Shakira, Gemma Arterton

3 Gertrude Stein, Isla Fisher, Amal Clooney

4 Charles Lindbergh, Rosa Parks, Betty Friedan, Alice Cooper, Natalie Imbruglia, Dara O'Briain

5 William Burroughs, Charlotte Rampling, Tom Wilkinson, Laura Linney, Hank Aaron, Jennifer Jason Leigh, Cristiano Ronaldo, Ben Ainslie, Michael Sheen, Bobby Brown

6 Ronald Reagan, Babe Ruth, Zsa Zsa Gabor, Bob Marley, Axl Rose, Calum Best

7 Charles Dickens, James Spader, Eddie Izzard, Garth Brooks, Chris Rock, Ashton Kutcher

8 Jules Verne, Jack Lemmon, Lana Turner, Nick Nolte, James Dean, Trinny Woodall

9 Carmen Miranda, Alice Walker, Carole King, Joe Pesci, Mia Farrow, Travis Tritt, Erin O'Connor, Zhang Ziyi, Tom Hiddleston, Amber Valletta

10 Robert Wagner, Laura Dern, Holly Willoughby, Emma Roberts, Chloe Grace Moretz, Keeley Hawes

11 Thomas Edison, Mary Quant, Burt Reynolds, Sheryl Crow, Jennifer Aniston, Brandy Norwood, Natalie Dormer, Taylor Lautner, Kelly Rowland

12 Abraham Lincoln, Charles Darwin, Arsenio Hall, Patricia Field, Darren Aronofsky, Christina Ricci, Josh Brolin

13 Jerry Springer, Kim Novak, Oliver Reed, Peter Gabriel, Robbie Williams, Mena Suvari, Prince Michael Jackson Jr

14 Michael Bloomberg, Florence Henderson, Rob Thomas

15 Susan B. Anthony, Matt Groening, Jane Seymour, Janice Dickinson, Renee O'Connor

16 Eckhart Tolle, Sonny Bono, John McEnroe, Cathy Freeman, Amanda Holden, Valentino Rossi, Agyness Deyn, Mahershala Ali, The Weeknd, Ice-T, Elizabeth Olsen

17 Barry Humphries, Rene Russo, Michael Jordan, Dominic Purcell, Denise Richards, Jerry O'Connell, Paris Hilton, Ed Sheeran, Sasha Pieterse, Joseph Gordon-Levitt, Billie Joe Armstrong, Selita Ebanks

Yoko Ono, Toni Morrison, John Travolta, Cybill Shepherd, Greta Scacchi, Matt Dillon, Molly Ringwald, Prue Leith, Dr Dre

Q&A Section

• • • • •

Q. What is the difference between a Sun sign and a Star sign?

A. They are the same thing. The Sun spends one month in each of the twelve star signs every year, so if you were born on 1 January, you are a Sun Capricorn. In astronomy, the Sun is termed a star rather than a planet, which is why the two names are interchangeable. The term 'zodiac sign', too, means the same as Sun sign and Star sign and is another way of describing which one of the twelve star signs you are, e.g. Sun Capricorn.

Q. What does it mean if I'm born on the cusp?

A. Being born on the cusp means that you were born on a day when the Sun moves from one of the twelve zodiac signs into the next. However, the Sun doesn't change signs at the same time each year. Sometimes it can be a day earlier or a day later. In the celebrity birthday section of the book, names in brackets mean that this person's birthday falls into this category.

If you know your complete birth data, including the date, time and place you were born, you can find out definitively what Sun sign you are. You do this by either checking an ephemeris (a planetary table) or asking an astrologer. For example, if a baby were born on 20 January 2018, it would be Sun Capricorn if born before 03:09 GMT or Sun Aquarius if born after 03:09 GMT. A year earlier, the Sun left Capricorn a day earlier and entered Aquarius on 19 January 2017, at 21:24 GMT. Each year the time changes are slightly different.

Q. Has my sign of the zodiac changed since I was born?

A. Every now and again, the media talks about a new sign of the zodiac called Ophiuchus and about there now being thirteen signs. This means that you're unlikely to be the same Sun sign as you always thought you were.

This method is based on fixing the Sun's movement to the star constellations in the sky, and is called 'sidereal' astrology. It's used traditionally in India and other Asian countries.

The star constellations are merely namesakes for the twelve zodiac signs. In western astrology, the zodiac is divided into twelve equal parts that are in sync with the seasons. This method is called 'tropical' astrology. The star constellations and the zodiac signs aren't the same.

Astrology is based on a beautiful pattern of symmetry (see Additional Information) and it wouldn't be the same if a thirteenth sign were introduced into the pattern. So never fear, no one is going to have to say their star sign is Ophiuchus, a name nobody even knows how to pronounce!

Q. Is astrology still relevant to me if I was born in the southern hemisphere?

A. Yes, astrology is unquestionably relevant to you. Astrology's origins, however, were founded in the northern hemisphere, which is why the Spring Equinox coincides with the Sun's move into Aries, the first sign of the zodiac. In the southern hemisphere, the seasons are reversed. Babylonian, Egyptian and Greek and Roman astrology are the forebears of modern-day astrology, and all of these civilisations were located in the northern hemisphere.

• • • • •

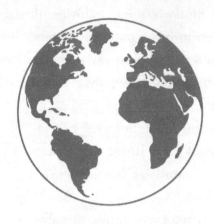

Q. Should I read my Sun sign, Moon sign and Ascendant sign?

A. If you know your horoscope or you have drawn up an astrology wheel for the time of your birth, you will be aware that you are more than your Sun sign. The Sun is the most important star in the sky, however, because the other planets revolve around it, and your horoscope in the media is based on Sun signs. The Sun represents your essence, who you are striving to become throughout your lifetime.

The Sun, Moon and Ascendant together give you a broader impression of yourself as all three reveal further elements about your personality. If you know your Moon and Ascendant signs, you can read all three books to gain further insight into who you are. It's also a good idea to read the Sun sign book that relates to your partner, parents, children, best friends, even your boss for a better understanding of their characters too.

Q. Is astrology a mix of fate and free will?

A. Yes. Astrology is not causal, i.e. the planets don't cause things to happen in your life; instead, the two are interconnected, hence the saying 'As above, so below'. The symbolism of the planets' movements mirrors what's happening on earth and in your personal experience of life.

You can choose to sit back and let your life unfold, or you can decide the best course of action available to you. In this way, you are combining your fate and free will, and this is one of astrology's major purposes in life. A knowledge of astrology can help you live more authentically, and it offers you a fresh perspective on how best to make progress in your life.

Q. What does it mean if I don't identify with my Sun sign? Is there a reason for this?

A. The majority of people identify with their Sun sign, and it is thought that one route to fulfilment is to grow into your Sun sign. You do get the odd exception, however.

For example, a Pisces man was adamant that he wasn't at all romantic, mystical, creative or caring, all typical Pisces archetypes. It turned out he'd spent the whole of his adult life working in the oil industry and lived primarily on the sea. Neptune is one of Pisces' ruling planets and god of the sea and Pisces rules all liquids, including oil. There's the Pisces connection.

Q. What's the difference between astrology and astronomy?

A. Astrology means 'language of the stars', whereas astronomy means 'mapping of the stars'. Traditionally, they were considered one discipline, one form of study and they coexisted together for many hundreds of years. Since the dawn of the Scientific Age, however, they have split apart.

Astronomy is the scientific strand, calculating and logging the movement of the planets, whereas astrology is the interpretation of the movement of the stars. Astrology works on a symbolic and intuitive level to offer guidance and insight. It reunites you with a universal truth, a knowingness that can sometimes get lost in place of an objective, scientific truth. Both are of value.

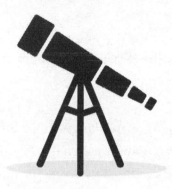

Q. What is a cosmic marriage in astrology?

A. One of the classic indicators of a relationship that's a match made in heaven is the union of the Sun and Moon. When they fall close to each other in the same sign in the birth charts of you and your partner, this is called a cosmic marriage. In astrology, the Sun and Moon are the king and queen of the heavens; the Sun is a masculine energy, and the Moon a feminine energy. They represent the eternal cycle of day and night, yin and yang.

Q. What does the Saturn Return mean?

A. In traditional astrology, Saturn was the furthest planet from the Sun, representing boundaries and the end of the universe. Saturn is linked to karma and time, and represents authority, structure and responsibility. It takes Saturn twenty-nine to thirty years to make a complete cycle of the zodiac and return to the place where it was when you were born.

This is what people mean when they talk about their Saturn Return; it's the astrological coming of age. Turning thirty can be a soul-searching time, when you examine how far you've come in life and whether you're on the right track. It's a watershed moment, a reality check and a defining stage of adulthood. The decisions you make during your Saturn Return are crucial, whether they represent endings or new commitments. Either way, it's the start of an important stage in your life path.

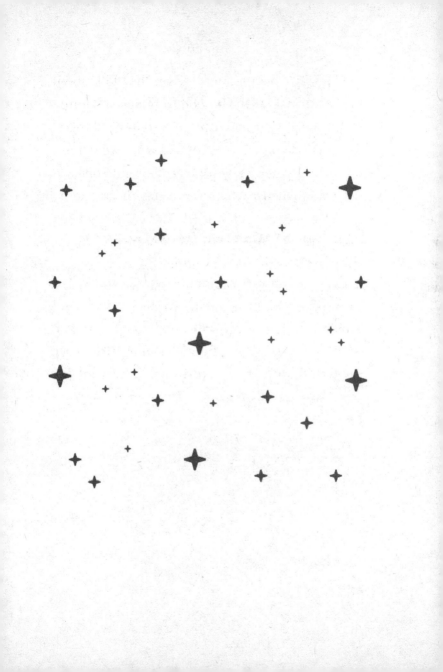

Additional Information

• • • • •

THE SYMMETRY OF ASTROLOGY

There is a beautiful symmetry to the zodiac (see horoscope wheel). There are twelve zodiac signs, which can be divided into two sets of 'introvert' and 'extrovert' signs, four elements (fire, earth, air, water), three modes (cardinal, fixed, mutable) and six pairs of opposite signs.

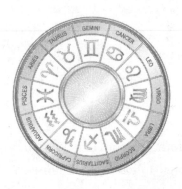

One of the values of astrology is in bringing opposites together, showing how they complement each other and work together and, in so doing, restore unity. The horoscope wheel represents the cyclical nature of life.

Aries (*March 21–April 19*)
Taurus (*April 20–May 20*)
Gemini (*May 21–June 20*)
Cancer (*June 21–July 22*)
Leo (*July 23–August 22*)
Virgo (*August 23 September 22*)
Libra (*September 23–October 23*)
Scorpio (*October 24–November 22*)
Sagittarius (*November 23–December 21*)
Capricorn (*December 22–January 20*)
Aquarius (*January 21–February 18*)
Pisces (*February 19–March 20*)

ELEMENTS

There are four elements in astrology and three signs allocated to each. The elements are:

fire – Aries, Leo, Sagittarius
earth – Taurus, Virgo, Capricorn
air – Gemini, Libra, Aquarius
water – Cancer, Scorpio, Pisces

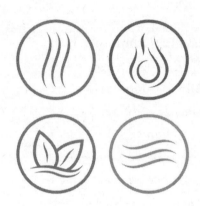

What each element represents:

Fire – fire blazes bright and fire types are inspirational, motivational, adventurous and love creativity and play

Earth – earth is grounding and solid, and earth rules money, security, practicality, the physical body and slow living

Air – air is intangible and vast and air rules thinking, ideas, social interaction, debate and questioning

Water – water is deep and healing and water rules feelings, intuition, quietness, relating, giving and sharing

MODES

There are three modes in astrology and four star signs allocated to each. The modes are:

cardinal – Aries, Cancer, Libra, Capricorn
fixed – Taurus, Leo, Scorpio, Aquarius
mutable – Gemini, Virgo, Sagittarius, Pisces

What each mode represents:

Cardinal – The first group represents the leaders of the zodiac, and these signs love to initiate and take action. Some say they're controlling.

Fixed – The middle group holds fast and stands the middle ground and acts as a stable, reliable companion. Some say they're stubborn.

Mutable – The last group is more willing to go with the flow and let life drift. They're more flexible and adaptable and often dual-natured. Some say they're all over the place.

INTROVERT AND EXTROVERT SIGNS/ OPPOSITE SIGNS

The introvert signs are the earth and water signs and the extrovert signs are the fire and air signs. Both sets oppose each other across the zodiac.

The 'introvert' earth and water oppositions are:

- Taurus – • Scorpio
- Cancer – • Capricorn
- Virgo – • Pisces

The 'extrovert' air and fire oppositions are:

- Aries – • Libra
- Gemini – • Sagittarius
- Leo – • Aquarius

THE HOUSES

The houses of the astrology wheel are an additional component to Sun sign horoscopes. The symmetry that is inherent within astrology remains, as the wheel is divided into twelve equal sections, called 'houses'. Each of the twelve houses is governed by one of the twelve zodiac signs.

There is an overlap in meaning as you move round the houses. Once you know the symbolism of all the star signs, it can be fleshed out further by learning about the areas of life represented by the twelve houses.

The houses provide more specific information if you choose to have a detailed birth chart reading.

This is based not only on your day of birth, which reveals your star sign, but also your time and place of birth. Here's the complete list of the meanings of the twelve houses and the zodiac sign they are ruled by:

1 – **Aries:** self, physical body, personal goals

2 – **Taurus:** money, possessions, values

3 – **Gemini:** communication, education, siblings, local neighbourhood

4 – **Cancer:** home, family, roots, the past, ancestry

5 – **Leo:** creativity, romance, entertainment, children, luck

6 – **Virgo:** work, routine, health, service

7 – **Libra:** relationships, the 'other', enemies, contracts

8 – **Scorpio:** joint finances, other people's resources, all things hidden and taboo

9 – **Sagittarius:** travel, study, philosophy, legal affairs, publishing, religion

10 – **Capricorn:** career, vocation, status, reputation

11 – **Aquarius:** friends, groups, networks, social responsibilities

12 – **Pisces:** retreat, sacrifice, spirituality

A GUIDE TO LOVE MATCHES

The star signs relate to each other in different ways depending on their essential nature. It can also be helpful to know the pattern they create across the zodiac. Here's a quick guide that relates to the chapter on Love Matches:

Two Peas In A Pod – the same star sign

Opposites Attract – star signs opposite each other

Soulmates – five or seven signs apart, and a traditional 'soulmate' connection

In Your Element – four signs apart, which means you share the same element

Squaring Up To Each Other – three signs apart, which means you share the same mode

Sexy Sextiles – two signs apart, which means you're both 'introverts' or 'extroverts'

Next Door Neighbours – one sign apart, different in nature but often share close connections